Best Keto Diet Cookbook

The Best Tasty Ketogenic Diet Recipes, Quick Meals Ready In 30 Minutes Or Less for Lose Weight in Health

Tanya Scofield

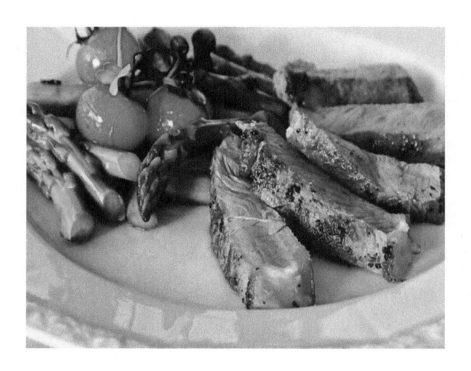

Table of Contents

consent from the Publisher. All additional right reserved.

The information in the following pages is broadly considered a truthful and accurate account of facts and as such, any inattention, use, or misuse of the information in question by the reader will render any resulting actions solely under their purview. There are no scenarios in which the publisher or the original author of this work can be in any fashion deemed liable for any hardship or damages that may befall them after undertaking information described herein.

Additionally, the information in the following pages is intended only for informational purposes and should thus be thought of as universal. As befitting its nature, it is presented without assurance regarding its prolonged validity or interim quality. Trademarks that are mentioned are done without written consent and can in no way be considered an endorsement from the trademark holder.

INTRODUCTION

So the Ketogenic Diet is all about reducing the amount of carbohydrates you eat. Does this mean you won't get the kind of energy you need for the day? Of course not! It only means that now, your body has to find other possible sources of energy. Do you know where they will be getting that energy? Even before we talk about how to do keto – it's important to first consider why this particular diet works. What actually happens to your body to make you lose weight? As you probably know, the body uses food as an energy source. Everything you eat is turned into energy, so that you can get up and do whatever you need to accomplish for the day. The main energy source is sugar so what happens is that you eat something, the body breaks it down into sugar, and the sugar is processed into energy. Typically, the "sugar" is taken directly from the food you eat so if you eat just the right amount of food, then your body is fueled for the whole day. If you eat too much, then the sugar is stored in your body – hence the accumulation of fat.

But what happens if you eat less food? This is where the Ketogenic Diet comes in. You see, the process of creating sugar from food is usually faster if the food happens to be rich in carbohydrates. Bread, rice, grain, pasta – all of these are carbohydrates and they're the easiest food types to turn into energy.

So here's the situation – you are eating less carbohydrates every day. To keep you energetic, the body breaks down the stored fat and turns them into molecules called ketone bodies. The process of turning the fat into ketone bodies is called "Ketosis" and obviously – this is where the name of the Ketogenic Diet comes from. The ketone bodies take the place of glucose in keeping you energetic. As long as you keep your carbohydrates reduced, the body will keep getting its energy from your body fat.

The Ketogenic Diet is often praised for its simplicity and when you look at it properly, the process is really straightforward. The Science behind the effectivity of the diet is also well-documented, and has been proven multiple times by different medical fields. For example, an article on Diet Review by Harvard provided a lengthy discussion on how the Ketogenic Diet works and why it is so effective for those who choose to use this diet.

But Fat Is the Enemy...Or Is It?

No – fat is NOT the enemy. Unfortunately, years of bad science told us that fat is something you have to avoid – but it's actually a very helpful thing for weight loss! Even before we move forward with this book, we'll have to discuss exactly what "healthy fats" are, and why they're actually the good guys. To do this, we need to make a distinction between the different kinds of fat. You've probably heard of them before and it is a little bit confusing at first. We'll try to go through them as simply as possible:

Saturated fat. This is the kind you want to avoid. They're also called "solid fat" because each molecule is packed with hydrogen atoms. Simply put, it's the kind of fat that can easily cause a blockage in your body. It can raise cholesterol levels and lead to heart problems or a stroke. Saturated fat is something you can find in meat, dairy products, and other processed food items. Now, you're probably wondering: isn't the Ketogenic Diet packed with saturated fat? The answer is: not necessarily. You'll find later in the recipes given that the Ketogenic Diet promotes primarily unsaturated fat or healthy fat. While there are definitely many meat recipes in the list, most of these recipes contain healthy fat sources.

Unsaturated Fat. These are the ones dubbed as healthy fat. They're the kind of fat you find in avocado, nuts, and other ingredients you usually find in Keto-friendly recipes. They're known to lower blood cholesterol and actually come in two types: polyunsaturated and monounsaturated. Both are good for your body but the benefits slightly vary, depending on what you're consuming.

Crab Cakes

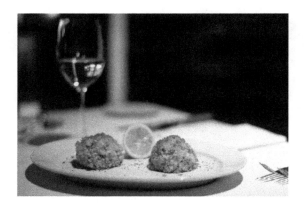

Preparation Time: 1 hour and 20 minutes

Cooking Time: 20 minutes

Servings: 8

Ingredients:

- 2 tablespoons butter
- 2 cloves garlic, minced
- ½ cup bell pepper, chopped
- 1 rib celery, chopped
- 1 shallot, chopped
- Salt and pepper to taste
- 2 tablespoons mayonnaise
- 1 egg, beaten
- 1 teaspoon mustard
- 1 tablespoon Worcestershire sauce

- 1 teaspoon hot sauce
- ½ cup Parmesan cheese, grated
- ½ cup pork rinds, crushed
- 1 lb. crabmeat
- 2 tablespoons olive oil

Directions:

- Add the butter to the pan over medium heat.
- Add the garlic, bell pepper, celery, shallot, salt and pepper.
- Cook for 10 minutes.
- In a bowl, mix the mayo, egg, Worcestershire, mustard and hot sauce.
- Add the sautéed vegetables to this mixture.
- Mix well.
- Add the cheese and pork rind.
- Fold in the crabmeat.
- Line the baking sheet with foil.
- Create patties from the mixture.
- Place the patties on the baking sheet.
- Cover the baking sheet with foil.
- Refrigerate for 1 hour.
- Fry in olive oil in a pan over medium heat.
- Cook until crispy and golden brown.

Nutrition: Calories 150 Total Fat 9.2g Saturated Fat 3.2g Cholesterol 43mg Sodium 601mg Total Carbohydrate 10.8g Dietary Fiber 0.5gTotal Sugars 4.6g Protein 6.4g Potassium 80mg

Tuna Salad

Preparation Time: 5 minutes

Cooking Time: 0 minute

Servings: 2

Ingredients:

- 1 cup tuna flakes
- 3 tablespoons mayonnaise
- 1 teaspoon onion flakes
- Salt and pepper to taste
- 3 cups Romaine lettuce

Directions:

1. Mix the tuna flakes, mayonnaise, onion flakes, salt and pepper in a bowl.
2. Serve with lettuce.

Nutrition: Calories 130 Total Fat 7.8g Saturated Fat 1.1g Cholesterol 13mg Sodium 206mg
Total Carbohydrate 8.5g Dietary Fiber 0.6g Total Sugars 2.6g Protein 8.2g Potassium 132mg

Keto Frosty

Preparation Time: 45 minutes

Cooking Time: 0 minute

Servings: 4

Ingredients:

- 1 ½ cups heavy whipping cream
- 2 tablespoons cocoa powder (unsweetened)
- 3 tablespoons Swerve
- 1 teaspoon pure vanilla extract
- Salt to taste

Directions:

1. In a bowl, combine all the ingredients.
2. Use a hand mixer and beat until you see stiff peaks forming.
3. Place the mixture in a Ziploc bag.
4. Freeze for 35 minutes.
5. Serve in bowls or dishes.

Nutrition:

Calories 164

Total Fat 17g

Saturated Fat 10.6g

Cholesterol 62mg

Sodium 56mg

Total Carbohydrate 2.9g

Dietary Fiber 0.8g

Total Sugars 0.2g

Protein 1.4g

Potassium 103mg

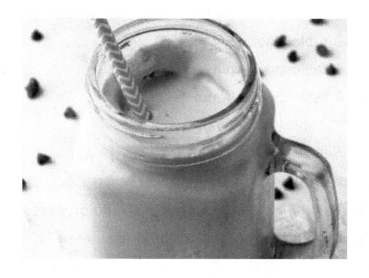

Keto Shake

Preparation Time: 15 minutes

Cooking Time: 0 minute

Serving: 1

Ingredients:

- ¾ cup almond milk
- ½ cup ice
- 2 tablespoons almond butter
- 2 tablespoons cocoa powder (unsweetened)
- 2 tablespoons Swerve
- 1 tablespoon chia seeds
- 2 tablespoons hemp seeds
- ½ tablespoon vanilla extract
- Salt to taste

Directions:

1. Blend all the ingredients in a food processor.
2. Chill in the refrigerator before serving.

Nutrition: Calories 104 Total Fat 9.5g Saturated Fat 5.1g Cholesterol 0mg Sodium 24mg Total Carbohydrate 3.6g Dietary Fiber 1.4g Total Sugars 1.1g Protein 2.9g Potassium 159mg

Keto Fat Bombs

Preparation Time: 30 minutes

Cooking Time: 0 minute

Servings: 10

Ingredients:

- 8 tablespoons butter
- ¼ cup Swerve
- ½ teaspoon vanilla extract
- Salt to taste
- 2 cups almond flour
- 2/3 cup chocolate chips

Directions:

1. In a bowl, beat the butter until fluffy.
2. Stir in the sugar, salt and vanilla.
3. Mix well.
4. Add the almond flour.
5. Fold in the chocolate chips.
6. Cover the bowl with cling wrap and refrigerate for 20 minutes.
7. Create balls from the dough.

Nutrition: Calories 176 Total Fat 15.2g Saturated Fat 8.4g Cholesterol 27mg Sodium 92mg Total Carbohydrate 12.9g Dietary Fiber 1g Total Sugars 10.8g Protein 2.2g Potassium 45mg

Avocado Ice Pops

Preparation Time: 20 minutes

Cooking Time: 0 minute

Servings: 10

Ingredients:

- 3 avocados
- ¼ cup lime juice
- 3 tablespoons Swerve
- ¾ cup coconut milk
- 1 tablespoon coconut oil
- 1 cup keto friendly chocolate

Directions:

1. Add all the ingredients except the oil and chocolate in a blender.
2. Blend until smooth.
3. Pour the mixture into the popsicle mold.
4. Freeze overnight.
5. In a bowl, mix oil and chocolate chips.
6. Melt in the microwave. And then let cool.
7. Dunk the avocado popsicles into the chocolate before serving.

Nutrition: Calories 176 Total Fat 17.4g Saturated Fat 7.5g Cholesterol 0mg Sodium 6mg

Total Carbohydrate 10.8g Dietary Fiber 4.5g Total
Sugars 5.4g Protein 1.6g Potassium 341mg

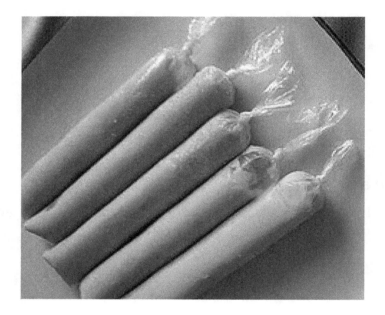

Carrot Balls

Preparation Time: 1 hour and 10 minutes

Cooking Time: 0 minute

Servings: 8

Ingredients:

- 8 oz. block cream cheese
- ¾ cup coconut flour
- ½ teaspoon pure vanilla extract
- 1 teaspoon stevia
- ¼ teaspoon ground nutmeg
- 1 teaspoon cinnamon
- 1 cup carrots, grated
- 1/2 cup pecans, chopped
- 1 cup coconut, shredded

Directions:

Use a hand mixer to beat the cream cheese, coconut flour, vanilla, stevia, nutmeg and cinnamon.

Fold in the carrots and pecans.

Form into balls.

Refrigerate for 1 hour.

Roll into shredded coconut before serving.

Nutrition: Calories 390 Total Fat 35g Saturated Fat 17g Cholesterol 60mg Sodium 202mg Total Carbohydrate 17.2g Dietary Fiber 7.8g Total Sugars 6g Protein 7.8g Potassium 154mg

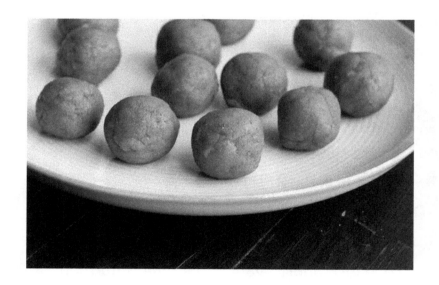

Coconut Crack Bars

Preparation Time: 2 minutes

Cooking Time: 3 minutes

Servings: 20

Ingredients:

- 3 cups coconut flakes (unsweetened)
- 1 cup coconut oil
- ¼ cup maple syrup

Directions:

1. Line a baking sheet with parchment paper.
2. Put coconut in a bowl.
3. Add the oil and syrup.
4. Mix well.
5. Pour the mixture into the pan.
6. Refrigerate until firm.
7. Slice into bars before serving.

Nutrition: Calories 147 Total Fat 14.9g Saturated Fat 13g Cholesterol 0mg Sodium 3mg

Total Carbohydrate 4.5g Dietary Fiber 1.1g Total Sugars 3.1g Protein 0.4g Potassium 51mg

Strawberry Ice Cream

Preparation Time: 1 hour and 20 minutes

Cooking Time: 0 minute

Servings: 4

Ingredients:

- 17 oz. coconut milk
- 16 oz. frozen strawberries
- ¾ cup Swerve
- ½ cup fresh strawberries

Directions:

1. Put all the ingredients except fresh strawberries in a blender.
2. Pulse until smooth.
3. Put the mixture in an ice cream maker.
4. Use ice cream maker according to directions.
5. Add the fresh strawberries a few minutes before the ice cream is done.
6. Freeze for 1 hour before serving.

Nutrition: Calories 320 Total Fat 28.8g Saturated Fat 25.5g Cholesterol 0mg Sodium 18mg Total Carbohydrate 25.3g Dietary Fiber 5.3g Total Sugars 19.1g Protein 2.9g Potassium 344mg

Key Lime Pudding

Preparation Time: 20 minutes

Cooking Time: 1 hour and 15 minutes

Servings: 2

Ingredients:

- 1 cup hot water
- 2/4 cup erythrytol syrup
- 6 drops stevia
- 1 teaspoon almond extract
- 1 teaspoon vanilla extract
- ¼ teaspoon Xanthan gum powder
- 2 ripe avocados, sliced
- 1 ½ oz. lime juice
- 3 tablespoons coconut oil
- Salt to taste

Directions:

1. Add water, erythritol, stevia, almond extract and vanilla extract to a pot.
2. Bring to a boil.
3. Simmer until the syrup has been reduced and has thickened.
4. Turn the heat off.
5. Add the gum powder.

6. Mix until thickened.

7. Add the avocado into a food processor.

8. Add the rest of the ingredients.

9. Pulse until smooth.

10. Place the mixture in ramekins.

11. Refrigerate for 1 hour.

12. Pour the syrup over the pudding before serving.

Nutrition: Calories 299 Total Fat 29.8g Saturated Fat 12.9g Cholesterol 0mg Sodium 47mg Total Carbohydrate 9.7g Dietary Fiber 6.8g Total Sugars 0.8g Protein 2g Potassium 502mg

Chicken, Bacon and Avocado Cloud Sandwiches

Preparation Time: 10 minutes

Cooking Time: 25 minutes

Servings: 6

Ingredients:

- For cloud bread
- 3 large eggs
- 4 oz. cream cheese
- ½ tablespoon. ground psyllium husk powder
- ½ teaspoon baking powder
- A pinch of salt
- To assemble sandwich
- 6 slices of bacon, cooked and chopped
- 6 slices pepper Jack cheese
- ½ avocado, sliced
- 1 cup cooked chicken breasts, shredded
- 3 tablespoons. mayonnaise

Directions:

1. Preheat your oven to 300 degrees.
2. Prepare a baking sheet by lining it with parchment paper.

3. Separate the egg whites and egg yolks, and place into separate bowls.

4. Whisk the egg whites until very stiff. Set aside.

5. Combined egg yolks and cream cheese.

6. Add the psyllium husk powder and baking powder to the egg yolk mixture. Gently fold in.

7. Add the egg whites into the egg mixture and gently fold in.

8. Dollop the mixture onto the prepared baking sheet to create 12 cloud bread. Use a spatula to gently spread the circles around to form ½-inch thick pieces.

9. Bake for 25 minutes or until the tops are golden brown.

10.Allow the cloud bread to cool completely before serving. Can be refrigerated for up to 3 days of frozen for up to 3 months. If food prepping, place a layer of parchment paper between each bread slice to avoid having them getting stuck together. Simply toast in the oven for 5 minutes when it is time to serve.

11.To assemble sandwiches, place mayonnaise on one side of one cloud bread. Layer with the remaining sandwich ingredients and top with another slice of cloud bread.

Nutrition: Calories: 333 kcal Carbs: 5g Fat: 26g Protein: 19.9g

Roasted Lemon Chicken Sandwich

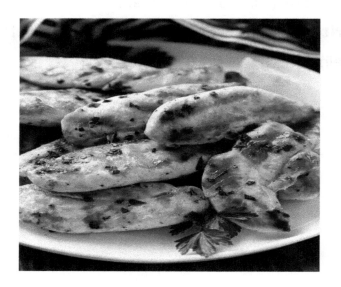

Preparation Time: 15 minutes

Cooking Time: 1 hour 30 minutes

Servings: 12

Ingredients:

- 1 kg whole chicken
- 5 tablespoons. butter
- 1 lemon, cut into wedges
- 1 tablespoon. garlic powder
- Salt and pepper to taste
- 2 tablespoons. mayonnaise
- Keto-friendly bread

Directions:

1. Preheat the oven to 350 degrees F.
2. Grease a deep baking dish with butter.
3. Ensure that the chicken is patted dry and that the gizzards have been removed.
4. Combine the butter, garlic powder, salt and pepper.
5. Rub the entire chicken with it, including in the cavity.
6. Place the lemon and onion inside the chicken and place the chicken in the prepared baking dish.
7. Bake for about 1½ hours, depending on the size of the chicken.
8. Baste the chicken often with the drippings. If the drippings begin to dry, add water. The chicken is done when a thermometer, insert it into the thickest part of the thigh reads 165 degrees F or when the clear juices run when the thickest part of the thigh is pierced.
9. Allow the chicken to cool before slicing.
10. To assemble sandwich, shred some of the breast meat and mix with the mayonnaise. Place the mixture between the two bread slices.

11.To save the chicken, refrigerated for up to 5 days or freeze for up to 1 month.

Nutrition: Calories: 214 kcal Carbs: 1.6 gFat: 11.8 gProtein: 24.4 g.

Keto-Friendly Skillet Pepperoni Pizza

Preparation Time: 10 minutes

Cooking Time: 6 minutes

Servings: 4

Ingredients:

- For Crust
- ½ cup almond flour
- ½ teaspoon baking powder
- 8 large egg whites, whisked into stiff peaks
- Salt and pepper to taste
- Toppings
- 3 tablespoons. Unsweetened tomato sauce
- ½ cup shredded cheddar cheese
- ½ cup pepperoni

Directions

1. Gently incorporate the almond flour into the egg whites. Ensure that no lumps remain.
2. Stir in the remaining crust ingredients.
3. Heat a nonstick skillet over medium heat. Spray with nonstick spray.

4. Pour the batter into the heated skillet to cover the bottom of the skillet.

5. Cover the skillet with a lid and cook the pizza crust to cook for about 4 minutes or until bubbles that appear on the top.

6. Flip the dough and add the toppings, starting with the tomato sauce and ending with the pepperoni

7. Cook the pizza for 2 more minutes.

8. Allow the pizza to cool slightly before serving.

9. Can be stored in the refrigerator for up to 5 days and frozen for up to 1 month.

Nutrition: Calories: 175 kcalCarbs: 1.9 g Fat: 12 gProtein: 14.3 g.

Cheesy Chicken Cauliflower

Preparation Time: 5 minutes

Cooking Time: 10 minutes

Servings: 4

Ingredients:

- 2 cups cauliflower florets, chopped
- ½ cup red bell pepper, chopped
- 1 cup roasted chicken, shredded (Lunch Recipes: Roasted Lemon Chicken Sandwich)
- ¼ cup shredded cheddar cheese
- 1 tablespoon. butter
- 1 tablespoon. sour cream
- Salt and pepper to taste

Directions:

1. Stir fry the cauliflower and peppers in the butter over medium heat until the veggies are tender.
2. Add the chicken and cook until the chicken is warmed through.
3. Add the remaining ingredients and stir until the cheese is melted.
4. Serve warm.

Nutrition: Calories: 144 kcal Carbs: 4 gFat: 8.5 gProtein: 13.2 g.

Chicken Soup

Preparation Time: 10 minutes

Cooking Time: 25 minutes

Servings: 6

Ingredients:

- 4 cups roasted chicken, shredded (Lunch Recipes: Roasted Lemon Chicken Sandwich)
- 2 tablespoons. butter
- 2 celery stalks, chopped
- 1 cup mushrooms, sliced
- 4 cups green cabbage, sliced into strips
- 2 garlic cloves, minced
- 6 cups chicken broth
- 1 carrot, sliced
- Salt and pepper to taste
- 1 tablespoon. garlic powder
- 1 tablespoon. onion powder

Directions:

1. Sauté the celery, mushrooms and garlic in the butter in a pot over medium heat for 4 minutes.
2. Add broth, carrots, garlic powder, onion powder, salt, and pepper.

3. Simmer for 10 minutes or until the vegetables are tender.

4. Add the chicken and cabbage and simmer for another 10 minutes or until the cabbage is tender.

5. Serve warm.

6. Can be refrigerated for up to 3 days or frozen for up to 1 month.

Nutrition: Calories: 279 kcal Carbs: 7.5 gFat: 12.3 g Protein: 33.4 g.

Chicken Avocado Salad

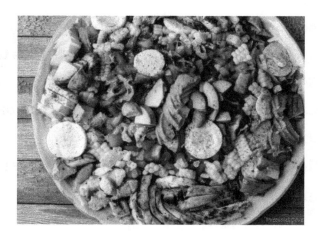

Preparation Time: 7 minutes

Cooking Time: 10 minutes

Servings: 4

Ingredients:

- 1 cup roasted chicken, shredded (Lunch Recipes: Roasted Lemon Chicken Sandwich)
- 1 bacon strip, cooked and chopped
- 1/2 medium avocado, chopped
- ¼ cup cheddar cheese, grated
- 1 hard-boiled egg, chopped
- 1 cup romaine lettuce, chopped
- 1 tablespoon. olive oil
- 1 tablespoon. apple cider vinegar

- Salt and pepper to taste

Directions:

1. Create the dressing by mixing apple cider vinegar, oil, salt and pepper.
2. Combine all the other ingredients in a mixing bowl.
3. Drizzle with the dressing and toss.
4. Can be refrigerated for up to 3 days.

Nutrition: Calories: 220 kcal Carbs: 2.8 g Fat: 16.7 gProtein: 14.8 g.

Chicken Broccoli Dinner

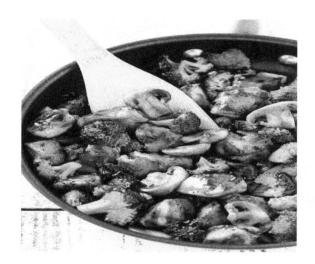

Preparation Time: 10 minutes

Cooking Time: 5 minutes

Servings: 1

Ingredients:

- 1 roasted chicken leg (Lunch Recipes: Roasted Lemon Chicken Sandwich)
- ½ cup broccoli florets
- ½ tablespoon. unsalted butter, softened
- 2 garlic cloves, minced
- Salt and pepper to taste

Directions:

1. Boil the broccoli in lightly salted water for 5 minutes. Drain the water from the pot and keep the broccoli in the pot. Keep the lid on to keep the broccoli warm.
2. Mix all the butter, garlic, salt and pepper in a small bowl to create garlic butter.
3. Place the chicken, broccoli and garlic butter.

Nutrition: Calories: 257 kcal Carbs: 5.1 g Fat: 14 gProtein: 27.4 g.

Easy Meatballs

Preparation Time: 10 minutes

Cooking Time: 20 minutes

Servings: 4

Ingredients:

- 1 lb. ground beef
- 1 egg, beaten
- Salt and pepper to taste
- 1 teaspoon garlic powder
- 1 teaspoon onion powder
- 2 tablespoons. butter
- ¼ cup mayonnaise
- ¼ cup pickled jalapeños
- 1 cup cheddar cheese, grated

Directions

1. Combine the cheese, mayonnaise, pickled jalapenos, salt, pepper, garlic powder and onion powder in a large mixing bowl.
2. Add the beef and egg and combine using clean hands.
3. Form large meatballs. Makes about 12.

4. Fry the meatballs in the butter over medium heat for about 4 minutes on each side or until golden brown.

5. Serve warm with a keto-friendly side.

6. The meatball mixture can also be used to make a meatloaf. Just preheat your oven to 400 degrees F, press the mixture into a loaf pan and bake for about 30 minutes or until the top is golden brown.

7. Can be refrigerated for up to 5 days or frozen for up to 3 months.

Nutrition: Calories: 454 kcalCarbs: 5 gFat: 28.2 gProtein: 43.2 g.

Chicken Casserole

Preparation Time: 10 minutes

Cooking Time: 40 minutes

Servings: 8

Ingredients:

- 1 lb. boneless chicken breasts, cut into 1" cubes
- 2 tablespoons. butter
- 4 tablespoons. green pesto
- 1 cup heavy whipping cream
- ¼ cup green bell peppers, diced
- 1 cup feta cheese, diced
- 1 garlic clove, minced
- Salt and pepper to taste

Directions

1. Preheat your oven to 400 degrees F.
2. Season the chicken with salt and pepper then batch fry in the butter until golden brown.
3. Place the fried chicken pieces in a baking dish. Add the feta cheese, garlic and bell peppers.
4. Combine the pesto and heavy cream in a bowl. Pour on top of the chicken mixture and spread with a spatula.

5. Bake for 30 minutes or until the casserole is light brown around the edges.
6. Serve warm.
7. Can be refrigerated for up to 5 days and frozen for 2 weeks.

Nutrition: Calories: 294 kcal Carbs: 1.7 g Fat: 22.7 g Protein: 20.1 g.

Lemon Baked Salmon

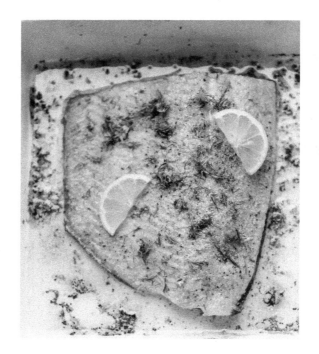

Preparation Time: 10 minutes

Cooking Time: 30 minutes

Servings: 4

Ingredients:

- 1 lb. salmon
- 1 tablespoon. olive oil
- Salt and pepper to taste
- 1 tablespoon. butter

- 1 lemon, thinly sliced
- 1 tablespoon. lemon juice

Directions:

1. Preheat your oven to 400 degrees F.
2. Grease a baking dish with the olive oil and place the salmon skin-side down.
3. Season the salmon with salt and pepper then top with the lemon slices.
4. Slice half the butter and place over the salmon.
5. Bake for 20minutes or until the salmon flakes easily.
6. Melt the remaining butter in a saucepan. When it starts to bubble, remove from heat and allow to cool before adding the lemon juice.
7. Drizzle the lemon butter over the salmon and Serve warm.

Nutrition: Calories: 211 kcal Carbs: 1.5 g Fat: 13.5 g Protein: 22.2 g.

Italian Sausage Stacks

Preparation Time: 10 minutes

Cooking Time: 25 minutes

Servings: 3

Ingredients:

- 6 Italian sausage patties
- 4 tablespoon olive oil
- 2 ripe avocados, pitted
- 2 teaspoon fresh lime juice
- Salt and black pepper to taste
- 6 fresh eggs
- Red pepper flakes to garnish

Directions:

1. In a skillet, warm the oil over medium heat and fry the sausage patties about 8 minutes until lightly browned and firm. Remove the patties to a plate.

2. Spoon the avocado into a bowl, mash with the lime juice, and season with salt and black pepper. Spread the mash on the sausages.

3. Boil 3 cups of water in a wide pan over high heat, and reduce to simmer (don't boil).

4. Crack each egg into a small bowl and gently put the egg into the simmering water; poach for 2 to 3 minutes. Use a perforated spoon to remove from the water on a paper towel to dry. Repeat with the other 5 eggs. Top each stack with a poached egg, sprinkle with chili flakes, salt, black pepper, and chives. Serve with turnip wedges.

Nutrition: Kcal 378, Fat 23g, Net Carbs 5g, Protein 16g

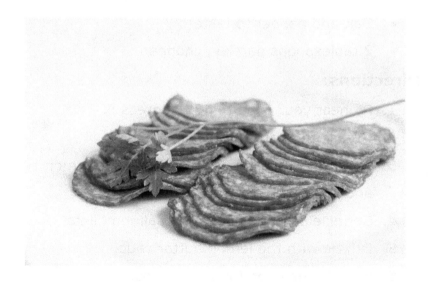

Baked Salmon

Preparation Time: 10 minutes

Cooking Time: 10 minutes

Servings: 4

Ingredients:

- Cooking spray
- 3 cloves garlic, minced
- ¼ cup butter
- 1 teaspoon lemon zest
- 2 tablespoons lemon juice
- 4 salmon fillets
- Salt and pepper to taste
- 2 tablespoons parsley, chopped

Directions:

1. Preheat your oven to 425 degrees F.
2. Grease the pan with cooking spray.
3. In a bowl, mix the garlic, butter, and lemon zest and lemon juice.
4. Sprinkle salt and pepper on salmon fillets.
5. Drizzle with the lemon butter sauce.
6. Bake in the oven for 12 minutes.
7. Garnish with parsley before serving.

Nutrition: Calories 345 Total Fat 22.7g Saturated Fat 8.9g Cholesterol 109mg Sodium 163mg Total Carbohydrate 1.2g Dietary Fiber 0.2g Total Sugars 0.2g Protein 34.9g Potassium 718mg

Tuna Patties

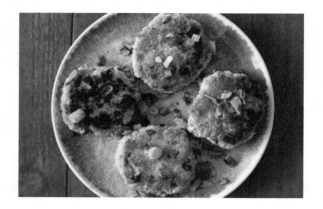

Preparation Time: 10 minutes

Cooking Time: 10 minutes

Servings: 8

Ingredients:

- 20 oz. canned tuna flakes
- ¼ cup almond flour
- 1 egg, beaten
- 2 tablespoons fresh dill, chopped
- 2 stalks green onion, chopped
- Salt and pepper to taste
- 1 tablespoon lemon zest
- ¼ cup mayonnaise
- 1 tablespoon lemon juice

- 2 tablespoons avocado oil

Directions:

1. Combine all the ingredients except avocado oil, lemon juice and avocado oil in a large bowl.
2. Form 8 patties from the mixture.
3. In a pan over medium heat, add the oil.
4. Once the oil starts to sizzle, cook the tuna patties for 3 to 4 minutes per side.
5. Drain each patty on a paper towel.
6. Spread mayo on top and drizzle with lemon juice before serving.

Nutrition: Calories 101 Total Fat 4.9g Saturated Fat 1.2g Cholesterol 47mg Sodium 243mg Total Carbohydrate 3.1g Dietary Fiber 0.5g Total Sugars 0.7g Protein 12.3g Potassium 60mg

Cauliflower Mash

Preparation Time: 10 minutes

Cooking Time: 5 minutes

Servings: 8

Ingredients:

- 4 cups cauliflower florets, chopped
- 1 cup grated parmesan cheese
- 6 tablespoons. butter
- ½ lemon, juice and zest
- Salt and pepper to taste

Directions:

1. Boil the cauliflower in lightly salted water over high heat for 5 minutes or until the florets are tender but still firm.
2. Strain the cauliflower in a colander and add the cauliflower to a food processor
3. Add the remaining ingredients and pulse the mixture to a smooth and creamy consistency
4. Serve with protein like salmon, chicken or meatballs.
5. Can be refrigerated for up to 3 days.

Nutrition: Calories: 101 kcal Carbs: 3.1 g Fat: 9.5 g Protein: 2.2 g.

Almond Waffles with Cinnamon Cream

Preparation Time: 10 minutes

Cooking Time: 25 minutes

Servings: 3

Ingredients:

- For the Spread
- 8 oz. cream cheese, at room temperature
- 1 teaspoon cinnamon powder
- 3 tablespoon swerve brown sugar
- Cinnamon powder for garnishing
- For the Waffles
- 5 tablespoon melted butter
- 1 ½ cups unsweetened almond milk
- 7 large eggs
- ¼ teaspoon liquid stevia
- ½ teaspoon baking powder
- 1 ½ cups almond flour

Directions:

1. Combine the cream cheese, cinnamon, and swerve with a hand mixer until smooth. Cover and chill until ready to use.

---

2. To make the waffles, whisk the butter, milk, and eggs in a medium bowl. Add the stevia and baking powder and mix. Stir in the almond flour and combine until no lumps exist. Let the batter sit for 5 minutes to thicken. Spritz a waffle iron with a non-stick cooking spray.

3. Ladle a ¼ cup of the batter into the waffle iron and cook according to the manufacturer's instructions until golden, about 10 minutes in total. Repeat with the remaining batter.

4. Slice the waffles into quarters; apply the cinnamon spread in between each of two waffles and snap. Sprinkle with cinnamon powder and serve.

Nutrition: Kcal 307, Fat 24g, Net Carbs 8g, Protein 12g

Grilled Mahi with Lemon Butter Sauce

Preparation Time: 20 minutes

Cooking Time: 10 minutes

Servings: 6

Ingredients:

- 6 mahi fillets
- Salt and pepper to taste
- 2 tablespoons olive oil
- 6 tablespoons butter
- ¼ onion, minced
- ½ teaspoon garlic, minced
- ¼ cup chicken stock
- 1 tablespoon lemon juice

Directions:

1. Preheat your grill to medium heat.
2. Season fish fillets with salt and pepper.
3. Coat both sides with olive oil.
4. Grill for 3 to 4 minutes per side.
5. Place fish on a serving platter.
6. In a pan over medium heat, add the butter and let it melt.

7. Add the onion and sauté for 2 minutes.

8. Add the garlic and cook for 30 seconds.

9. Pour in the chicken stock.

10. Simmer until the stock has been reduced to half.

11. Add the lemon juice.

12. Pour the sauce over the grilled fish fillets.

Nutrition: Calories 234 Total Fat 17.2g Saturated Fat 8.3g Cholesterol 117mg Sodium 242mg Total Carbohydrate 0.6g Dietary Fiber 0.1g Total Sugars 0.3g Protein 19.1g Potassium 385mg

Shrimp Scampi

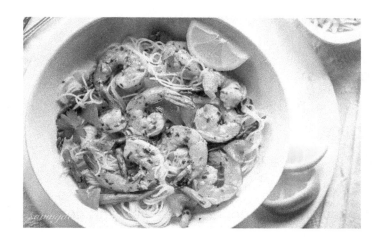

Preparation Time: 15 minutes

Cooking Time: 10 minutes

Servings: 6

Ingredients:

- 2 tablespoons olive oil
- 2 tablespoons butter
- 1 tablespoon garlic, minced
- ½ cup dry white wine
- ¼ teaspoon red pepper flakes
- Salt and pepper to taste

- 2 lb. large shrimp, peeled and deveined
- ¼ cup fresh parsley, chopped
- 1 teaspoon lemon zest
- 2 tablespoons lemon juice
- 3 cups spaghetti squash, cooked

Directions:

1. In a pan over medium heat, add the oil and butter.
2. Cook the garlic for 2 minutes.
3. Pour in the wine.
4. Add the red pepper flakes, salt and pepper.
5. Cook for 2 minutes.
6. Add the shrimp.
7. Cook for 2 to 3 minutes.
8. Remove from the stove.
9. Add the parsley, lemon zest and lemon juice.
10. Serve on top of spaghetti squash.

Nutrition: Calories 232 Total Fat 8.9g Saturated Fat 3.2g Cholesterol 226mg Sodium 229mg Total Carbohydrate 7.6g Dietary Fiber 0.2g Total Sugars 0.3g Protein 28.9g Potassium 104mg

Dark Chocolate Smoothie

Preparation Time: 10 minutes

Cooking Time: 25 minutes

Servings: 3

Ingredients:

- 8 pecans
- ¾ cup coconut milk
- ¼ cup water
- 1 ½ cups watercress
- 2 teaspoon vegan protein powder
- 1 tablespoon chia seeds
- 1 tablespoon unsweetened cocoa powder
- 4 fresh dates, pitted

Directions

1. In a blender, add all ingredients and process until creamy and uniform. Place into two glasses and chill before serving.

Nutrition: Kcal 335; Fat: 31.7g Net Carbs: 12.7g, Protein: 7g

Five Greens Smoothie

Preparation Time: 10 minutes

Cooking Time: 25 minutes

Servings: 3

Ingredients:

- 6 kale leaves, chopped
- 3 stalks celery, chopped
- 1 ripe avocado, skinned, pitted, sliced
- 1 cup ice cubes
- 2 cups spinach, chopped
- 1 large cucumber, peeled and chopped
- Chia seeds to garnish

Directions:

1. In a blender, add the kale, celery, avocado, and ice cubes, and blend for 45 seconds. Add the spinach and cucumber, and process for another 45 seconds until smooth.
2. Pour the smoothie into glasses, garnish with chia seeds and serve the drink immediately.

Nutrition: Kcal 124, Fat 7.8g, Net Carbs 2.9g, Protein 3.2g

Smoked Salmon Rolls with Dill Cream Cheese

Preparation Time: 10 minutes

Cooking Time: 25 minutes

Servings: 3

Ingredients:

- 3 tablespoon cream cheese, softened
- 1 small lemon, zested and juiced
- 3 teaspoon chopped fresh dill
- Salt and black pepper to taste
- 3 (7-inch) low carb tortillas
- 6 slices smoked salmon

Directions

1. In a bowl, mix the cream cheese, lemon juice, zest, dill, salt, and black pepper.
2. Lay each tortilla on a plastic wrap (just wide enough to cover the tortilla), spread with cream cheese mixture, and top each (one) with two salmon slices. Roll up the tortillas and secure both ends by twisting.

3. Refrigerate for 2 hours, remove plastic, cut off both ends of each wrap, and cut wraps into wheels.

Nutrition: Kcal 250, Fat 16g, Net Carbs 7g, Protein 18g

Pan-Seared Halibut with Citrus Butter Sauce

Preparation Time: 10 minutes

Cooking Time: 15 minutes

Servings: 3

Ingredients:

- 4 (5-ounce) halibut fillets, each about 1 inch thick
- Sea salt
- Freshly ground black pepper
- ¼ cup butter
- 2 teaspoons minced garlic
- 1 shallot, minced
- 3 tablespoons dry white wine
- 1 tablespoon freshly squeezed lemon juice
- 1 tablespoon freshly squeezed orange juice
- 2 teaspoons chopped fresh parsley
- 2 tablespoons olive oil

Directions:

1. Pat the fish dry with paper towels and then lightly season the fillets with salt and pepper. Set aside on a paper towel–lined plate.

---

2. Place a small saucepan over medium heat and melt the butter.

3. Sauté the garlic and shallot until tender, about 3 minutes.

4. Whisk in the white wine, lemon juice, and orange juice and bring the sauce to a simmer, cooking until it thickens slightly, about 2 minutes.

5. Remove the sauce from the heat and stir in the parsley; set aside.

6. Place a large skillet over medium-high heat and add the olive oil.

7. Panfry the fish until lightly browned and just cooked through, turning them over once, about 10 minutes in total.

8. Serve the fish immediately with a spoonful of sauce for each.

Nutrition: Calories: 319 Fat: 26g Protein: 22g Carbohydrates: 2g Fiber: 0g

Lemon Butter Chicken

Preparation Time: 10 minutes

Cooking Time: 40 minutes

Servings: 4

Ingredients:

- 4 bone-in, skin-on chicken thighs
- Sea salt
- Freshly ground black pepper
- 2 tablespoons butter, divided
- 2 teaspoons minced garlic
- ½ cup Herbed Chicken Stock
- ½ cup heavy (whipping) cream
- Juice of ½ lemon

Directions:

1. Preheat the oven to 400°F.
2. Lightly season the chicken thighs with salt and pepper.
3. Place a large ovenproof skillet over medium-high heat and add 1 tablespoon of butter.
4. Brown the chicken thighs until golden on both sides, about 6 minutes in total. Remove the thighs to a plate and set aside.

5. Add the remaining 1 tablespoon of butter and sauté the garlic until translucent, about 2 minutes.
6. Whisk in the chicken stock, heavy cream, and lemon juice.
7. Bring the sauce to a boil and then return the chicken to the skillet.
8. Place the skillet in the oven, covered, and braise until the chicken is cooked through, about 30 minutes.

Nutrition: Calories: 294 Fat: 26g Protein: 12g Carbohydrates: 4g Fiber: 1g

Simple Fish Curry

Preparation Time: 10 minutes

Cooking Time: 25 minutes

Servings: 4

Ingredients:

- 2 tablespoons coconut oil
- 1½ tablespoons grated fresh ginger
- 2 teaspoons minced garlic
- 1 tablespoon curry powder
- ½ teaspoon ground cumin
- 2 cups coconut milk
- 16 ounces firm white fish, cut into 1-inch chunks
- 1 cup shredded kale
- 2 tablespoons chopped cilantro

Directions:

1. Place a large saucepan over medium heat and melt the coconut oil.
2. Sauté the ginger and garlic until lightly browned, about 2 minutes.
3. Stir in the curry powder and cumin and sauté until very fragrant, about 2 minutes.
4. Stir in the coconut milk and bring the liquid to a boil.

5. Reduce the heat to low and simmer for about 5 minutes to infuse the milk with the spices.

6. Add the fish and cook until the fish is cooked through, about 10 minutes.

7. Stir in the kale and cilantro and simmer until wilted, about 2 minutes.

8. Serve.

Nutrition: Calories: 416 Fat: 31g Protein: 26g Carbohydrates: 5g Fiber: 1g

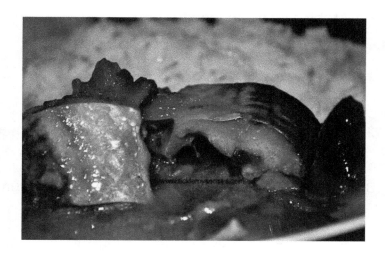

Roasted Salmon with Avocado Salsa

Preparation Time: 15 minutes

Cooking Time: 12 minutes

Servings: 4

Ingredients:

- For the Salsa
- 1 avocado, peeled, pitted, and diced
- 1 scallion, white and green parts, chopped
- ½ cup halved cherry tomatoes
- Juice of 1 lemon
- Zest of 1 lemon
- For the Fish
- 1 teaspoon ground cumin
- ½ teaspoon ground coriander
- ½ teaspoon onion powder
- ¼ teaspoon sea salt
- Pinch freshly ground black pepper
- Pinch cayenne pepper
- 4 (4-ounce) boneless, skinless salmon fillets
- 2 tablespoons olive oil

Directions:

1. To Make the Salsa
2. In a small bowl, stir together the avocado, scallion, tomatoes, lemon juice, and lemon zest until mixed.
3. Set aside.
4. To Make the Fish
5. Preheat the oven to 400°F. Line a baking sheet with aluminum foil and set aside.
6. In a small bowl, stir together the cumin, coriander, onion powder, salt, black pepper, and cayenne until well mixed.
7. Rub the salmon fillets with the spice mix and place them on the baking sheet.
8. Drizzle the fillets with the olive oil and roast the fish until it is just cooked through, about 15 minutes.
9. Serve the salmon topped with the avocado salsa.

Nutrition: Calories: 320 Fat: 26g Protein: 22g Carbohydrates: 4g Fiber: 3g

Sole Asiago

Preparation Time: 10 minutes

Cooking Time: 8 minutes

Servings: 4

Ingredients:

- 4 (4-ounce) sole fillets
- ¾ cup ground almonds
- ¼ cup Asiago cheese
- 2 eggs, beaten
- 2½ tablespoons melted coconut oil

Directions:

1. Preheat the oven to 350°F. Line a baking sheet with parchment paper and set aside.
2. Pat the fish dry with paper towels.
3. Stir together the ground almonds and cheese in a small bowl.
4. Place the bowl with the beaten eggs in it next to the almond mixture.
5. Dredge a sole fillet in the beaten egg and then press the fish into the almond mixture so it is completely coated. Place on the baking sheet and repeat until all the fillets are breaded.

6. Brush both sides of each piece of fish with the coconut oil.
7. Bake the sole until it is cooked through, about 8 minutes in total.
8. Serve immediately.

Nutrition: Calories: 406 Fat: 31g Protein: 29g Carbohydrates: 6g Fiber: 3g

Baked Coconut Haddock

Preparation Time: 10 minutes

Cooking Time: 12 minutes

Servings: 4

Ingredients:

- 4 (5-ounce) boneless haddock fillets
- Sea salt
- Freshly ground black pepper
- 1 cup shredded unsweetened coconut
- ¼ cup ground hazelnuts
- 2 tablespoons coconut oil, melted

Directions:

1. Preheat the oven to 400°F. Line a baking sheet with parchment paper and set aside.
2. Pat the fillets very dry with paper towels and lightly season them with salt and pepper.
3. Stir together the shredded coconut and hazelnuts in a small bowl.
4. Dredge the fish fillets in the coconut mixture so that both sides of each piece are thickly coated.
5. Place the fish on the baking sheet and lightly brush both sides of each piece with the coconut oil.

6. Bake the haddock until the topping is golden and the fish flakes easily with a fork, about 12 minutes total.

7. Serve.

8. PREP TIP the breading of the fish can be done ahead, up to 1 day, if you just want to pop the fish in the oven when you get home. Place the breaded fish on the baking sheet and cover it with plastic wrap in the refrigerator until you wish to bake it.

Nutrition: Calories: 299 Fat: 24g Protein: 20g Carbohydrates: 4g Fiber: 3g

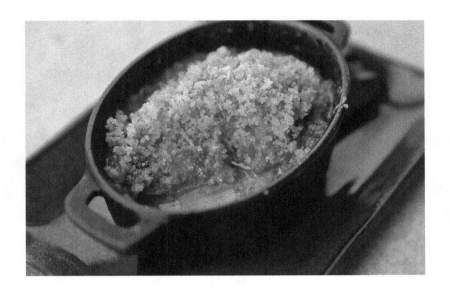

Cheesy Garlic Salmon

Preparation Time: 15 minutes

Cooking Time: 12 minutes

Servings: 4

Ingredients:

- ½ cup Asiago cheese
- 2 tablespoons freshly squeezed lemon juice
- 2 tablespoons butter, at room temperature
- 2 teaspoons minced garlic
- 1 teaspoon chopped fresh basil
- 1 teaspoon chopped fresh oregano
- 4 (5-ounce) salmon fillets
- 1 tablespoon olive oil

Directions:

1. Preheat the oven to 350°F. Line a baking sheet with parchment paper and set aside.

2. In a small bowl, stir together the Asiago cheese, lemon juice, butter, garlic, basil, and oregano.

3. Pat the salmon dry with paper towels and place the fillets on the baking sheet skin-side down. Divide the topping evenly between the fillets and spread it across the fish using a knife or the back of a spoon.

4. Drizzle the fish with the olive oil and bake until the topping is golden and the fish is just cooked through, about 12 minutes.

5. Serve.

Nutrition: Calories: 357 Fat: 28g Protein: 24g Carbohydrates: 2g Fiber: 0g

Chicken Bacon Burgers

Preparation Time: 10 minutes

Cooking Time: 25 minutes

Servings: 4

Ingredients:

- 1-pound ground chicken
- 8 bacon slices, chopped
- ¼ cup ground almonds
- 1 teaspoon chopped fresh basil
- ¼ teaspoon sea salt
- Pinch freshly ground black pepper
- 2 tablespoons coconut oil
- 4 large lettuce leaves
- 1 avocado, peeled, pitted, and sliced

Directions:

1. Preheat the oven to 350°F. Line a baking sheet with parchment paper and set aside.
2. In a medium bowl, combine the chicken, bacon, ground almonds, basil, salt, and pepper until well mixed.
3. Form the mixture into 6 equal patties.
4. Place a large skillet over medium-high heat and add the coconut oil.

5. Pan sear the chicken patties until brown on both sides, about 6 minutes in total.
6. Place the browned patties on the baking sheet and bake until completely cooked through, about 15 minutes.
7. Serve on the lettuce leaves, topped with the avocado slices.

Nutrition: Calories: 374 Fat: 33g Protein: 18g Carbohydrates: 3g Fiber: 2g

Herb Butter Scallops

Preparation Time: 10 minutes

Cooking Time: 10 minutes

Servings: 3

Ingredients:

- 1 pound sea scallops, cleaned
- Freshly ground black pepper
- 8 tablespoons butter, divided
- 2 teaspoons minced garlic
- Juice of 1 lemon
- 2 teaspoons chopped fresh basil
- 1 teaspoon chopped fresh thyme

Directions:

1. Pat the scallops dry with paper towels and season them lightly with pepper.
2. Place a large skillet over medium heat and add 2 tablespoons of butter.
3. Arrange the scallops in the skillet, evenly spaced but not too close together, and sear each side until they are golden brown, about 2½ minutes per side.
4. Remove the scallops to a plate and set aside.

5. Add the remaining 6 tablespoons of butter to the skillet and sauté the garlic until translucent, about 3 minutes.

6. Stir in the lemon juice, basil, and thyme and return the scallops to the skillet, turning to coat them in the sauce.

7. Serve immediately.

Nutrition: Calories: 306 Fat: 24g Protein: 19g Carbohydrates: 4g Fiber: 0g

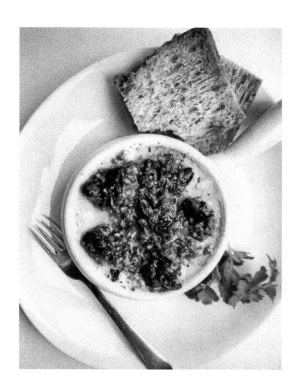

Paprika Chicken

Preparation Time: 10 minutes

Cooking Time: 25 minutes

Servings: 4

Ingredients:

- 4 (4-ounce) chicken breasts, skin-on
- Sea salt
- Freshly ground black pepper
- 1 tablespoon olive oil
- ½ cup chopped sweet onion
- ½ cup heavy (whipping) cream
- 2 teaspoons smoked paprika
- ½ cup sour cream
- 2 tablespoons chopped fresh parsley

Directions:

1. Lightly season the chicken with salt and pepper.
2. Place a large skillet over medium-high heat and add the olive oil.
3. Sear the chicken on both sides until almost cooked through, about 15 minutes in total. Remove the chicken to a plate.
4. Add the onion to the skillet and sauté until tender, about 4 minutes.

5. Stir in the cream and paprika and bring the liquid to a simmer.
6. Return the chicken and any accumulated juices to the skillet and simmer the chicken for 5 minutes until completely cooked.
7. Stir in the sour cream and remove the skillet from the heat.
8. Serve topped with the parsley.

Nutrition: Calories: 389 Fat: 30g Protein: 25g Carbohydrates: 4g Fiber: 0g

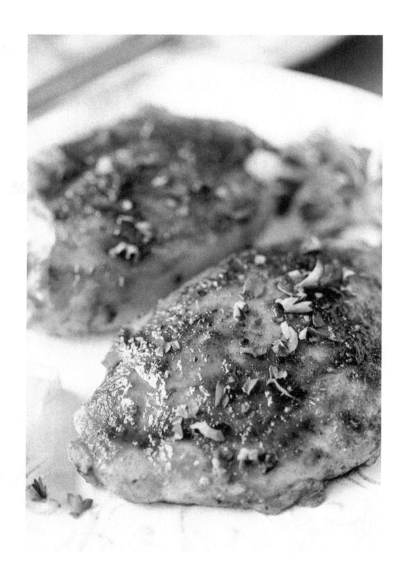

Trout and Chili Nuts

Preparation Time: 10 minutes

Cooking time: 0 minutes

Servings: 3

Ingredients:

- 1.5kg of rainbow trout
- 300gr shelled walnuts
- 1 bunch of parsley
- 9 cloves of garlic
- 7 tablespoons of olive oil
- 2 fresh hot peppers
- The juice of 2 lemons
- Halls

Directions:

1. Clean and dry the trout then place them in a baking tray.
2. Chop the walnuts, parsley and chili peppers then mash the garlic cloves.
3. Mix the ingredients by adding olive oil, lemon juice and a pinch of salt.
4. Stuff the trout with some of the sauce and use the rest to cover the fish.
5. Bake at 180° for 30/40 minutes.

6. Serve the trout hot or cold.

Nutrition: Calories 226 Fat 5 Fiber 2 Carbs 7 Protein 8

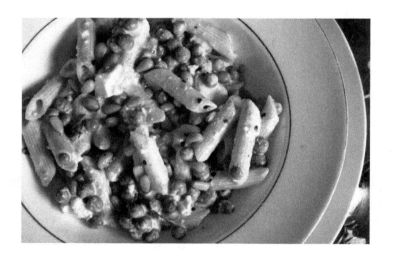

Nut Granola & Smoothie Bowl

Preparation Time: 10 minutes

Cooking time: 40 minutes

Servings: 3

Ingredients:

- 6 cups Greek yogurt
- 4 tablespoon almond butter
- A handful toasted walnuts
- 3 tablespoon unsweetened cocoa powder
- 4 teaspoon swerve brown sugar
- 2 cups nut granola for topping

Directions:

1. Combine the Greek yogurt, almond butter, walnuts, cocoa powder, and swerve brown sugar in a smoothie maker; puree in high-speed until smooth and well mixed.

2. Share the smoothie into four breakfast bowls, top with a half cup of granola each, and serve.

Nutrition: Kcal 361, Fat 31.2g, Net Carbs 2g, Protein 13g

Bacon and Egg Quesadillas

Preparation Time: 10 minutes

Cooking time: 30 minutes

Servings: 3

Ingredients:

- 8 low carb tortilla shells
- 6 eggs
- 1 cup water
- 3 tablespoon butter
- 1 ½ cups grated cheddar cheese
- 1 ½ cups grated Swiss cheese
- 5 bacon slices
- 1 medium onion, thinly sliced
- 1 tablespoon chopped parsley

Directions

1. Bring the eggs to a boil in water over medium heat for 10 minutes. Transfer the eggs to an ice water bath, peel the shells, and chop them; set aside.

2. Meanwhile, as the eggs cook, fry the bacon in a skillet over medium heat for 4 minutes until crispy. Remove and chop. Plate and set aside too.

3. Fetch out 2/3 of the bacon fat and sauté the onions in the remaining grease over medium heat for 2 minutesset aside. Melt 1 tablespoon of butter in a skillet over medium heat.

4. Lay one tortilla in a skillet; sprinkle with some Swiss cheese. Add some chopped eggs and bacon over the cheese, top with onion, and sprinkle with some cheddar cheese. Cover with another tortilla shell. Cook for 45 seconds, then carefully flip the quesadilla, and cook the other side too for 45 seconds. Remove to a plate and repeat the cooking process using the remaining tortilla shells.

5. Garnish with parsley and serve warm.

Nutrition: Kcal 449, Fat 48.7g, Net Carbs 6.8g, Protein 29.1g

Bacon and Cheese Frittata

Preparation Time: 10 minutes

Cooking time: 20 minutes

Servings: 3

Ingredients:

- 10 slices bacon
- 10 fresh eggs
- 3 tablespoon butter, melted
- ½ cup almond milk
- Salt and black pepper to taste
- 1 ½ cups cheddar cheese, shredded
- ¼ cup chopped green onions

Directions:

1. Preheat the oven to 400ºF and grease a baking dish with cooking spray. Cook the bacon in a skillet over medium heat for 6 minutes. Once crispy, remove from the skillet to paper towels and discard grease. Chop into small pieces. Whisk the eggs, butter, milk, salt, and black pepper. Mix in the bacon and pour the mixture into the baking dish.

2. Sprinkle with cheddar cheese and green onions, and bake in the oven for 10 minutes or until the

eggs are thoroughly cooked. Remove and cool the frittata for 3 minutes, slice into wedges, and serve warm with a dollop of Greek yogurt.

Nutrition: Kcal 325, Fat 28g, Net Carbs 2g, Protein 15g

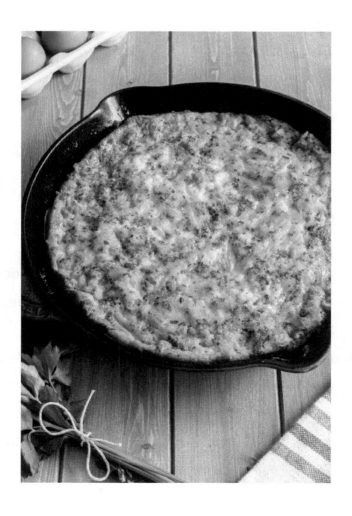

Spicy Egg Muffins with Bacon & Cheese

Preparation Time: 10 minutes

Cooking time: 20 minutes

Servings: 3

Ingredients:

- 12 eggs
- ¼ cup coconut milk
- Salt and black pepper to taste
- 1 cup grated cheddar cheese
- 12 slices bacon
- 4 jalapeño peppers, seeded and minced

Directions:

1. Preheat oven to 370ºF.
2. Crack the eggs into a bowl and whisk with coconut milk until combined. Season with salt and pepper, and evenly stir in the cheddar cheese.
3. Line each hole of a muffin tin with a slice of bacon and fill each with the egg mixture two-thirds way up. Top with the jalapeno peppers and bake in the oven for 18 to 20 minutes or until puffed and

golden. Remove, allow cooling for a few minutes, and serve with arugula salad.

Nutrition: Kcal 302, Fat 23.7g, Net Carbs 3.2g, Protein 20g

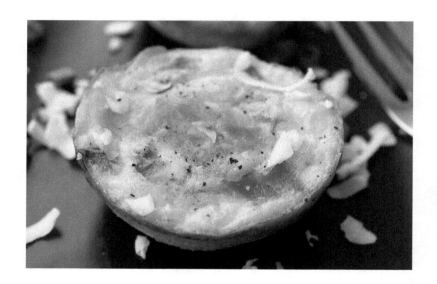

Ham & Egg Broccoli Bake

Preparation Time: 10 minutes

Cooking time: 25 minutes

Servings: 3

Ingredients:

- 2 heads broccoli, cut into small florets
- 2 red bell peppers, seeded and chopped
- ¼ cup chopped ham
- 2 teaspoon ghee
- 1 teaspoon dried oregano + extra to garnish
- Salt and black pepper to taste
- 8 fresh eggs

Directions

1. Preheat oven to 425ºF.

2. Melt the ghee in a frying pan over medium heat; brown the ham, stirring frequently, about 3 minutes.

3. Arrange the broccoli, bell peppers, and ham on a foil-lined baking sheet in a single layer, toss to combine; season with salt, oregano, and black pepper. Bake for 10 minutes until the vegetables have softened.

4. Remove, create eight indentations with a spoon, and crack an egg into each. Return to the oven and continue to bake for an additional 5 to 7 minutes until the egg whites are firm.

5. Season with salt, black pepper, and extra oregano, share the bake into four plates and serve with strawberry lemonade (optional).

Nutrition: Kcal 344, Fat 28g, Net Carbs 4.2g, Protein 11g

Hot Buffalo wings

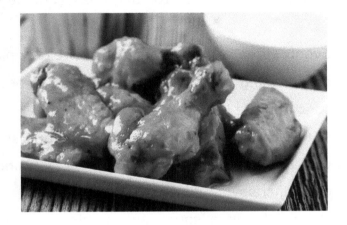

Preparation Time: 10 minutes

Cooking Time: 47 minutes

Servings: 3

Ingredients:

- Hot sauce ¼ cup
- Coconut oil 4 tablespoons, plus more for rubbing on the wings
- Chicken wings 12 (fresh or frozen)
- Garlic 1 clove, minced
- Salt ¼ teaspoon
- Paprika ¼ teaspoon
- Cayenne pepper ¼ teaspoon
- Ground black pepper 1 dash

Directions:

1. Preheat your oven to 400 degrees F (200 degrees C).

2. Evenly spread chicken wings on a wire rack placed on a baking dish (it will save wings to become soggy on the bottom).

3. Rub each chicken wing with olive oil and season with salt and pepper, then bake for 45 minutes, or until crispy.

4. Meanwhile, in a saucepan combine coconut oil and garlic and cook over medium heat for 1 minute, or until fragrant.

5. Remove from heat and stir in hot sauce, salt, paprika, cayenne pepper and black pepper.

6. Remove wings from the oven and transfer to a large bowl.

7. Pour hot sauce mixture over wings and toss until each wing is coated with the sauce.

8. Serve immediately.

Nutrition: Calories: 391 Carbohydrates: 1 g Fats: 33 g Protein: 31 g

Turkey Meatballs

Preparation Time: 30 minutes

Cooking Time: 0 minutes

Servings: 4

Ingredients:

- 255g turkey sausage
- 2 tablespoons of extra virgin olive oil
- One can of 425g chickpeas, rinsed and drained...
- 1/2 medium onion, chopped, 2/3 cup
- 2 cloves of garlic, finely chopped
- 1 teaspoon of cumin
- 1/2 cup flour
- 1/2 teaspoon instant yeast for desserts
- Salt and ground black pepper
- 1 cup of Greek yogurt
- 2 tablespoons of lime juice
- 2 radicchio hearts, chopped
- Hot sauce

Directions:

1. Preheat the oven to 200°C.
2. In a processor, blend the chickpeas, onion, garlic, cumin, 1 teaspoon salt and 1/2 teaspoon pepper until all the ingredients are finely chopped. Add

the flour, baking powder and blend to make everything mix well. Transfer to a medium bowl and add the sausage, stirring together with your hands. Cover and refrigerate for 30 minutes.

3. Once cold, take the mixture in spoonful, forming 1-inch balls with wet hands. Heat the olive oil in a pan over medium heat. In two groups, put the falafel in the pan and cook until slightly brown, about a minute and a half per side. Transfer to a baking tray and bake in the oven until well cooked, for about 10 minutes.

4. Mix together the yogurt, lime juice, 1/2 teaspoon salt and 1/4 teaspoon pepper. Divide the lettuce into 4 plates, season with some yogurt sauce.

Nutrition: Calories 189 Fat 5 Protein 77 Sugar 3

Chicken in Sweet and Sour Sauce with Corn Salad

Preparation Time: 10 minutes

Cooking Time: 15 minutes

Servings: 4

Ingredients:

- 2 cups plus 2 tablespoons of unflavored low-fat yoghurt
- 2 cups of frozen mango chunks
- 3 tablespoons of honey
- ¼ cup plus 1 tablespoon apple cider vinegar
- ¼ cup sultana
- 2 tablespoons of olive oil, plus an amount to be brushed
- ¼ teaspoon of cayenne pepper
- 5 dried tomatoes (not in oil)
- 2 small cloves of garlic, finely chopped
- 4 cobs, peeled
- 8 peeled and boned chicken legs, peeled (about 700g)
- Halls
- 6 cups of mixed salad

- 2 medium carrots, finely sliced

Directions:

1. For the smoothie: in a blender, mix 2 cups of yogurt, 2 cups of ice, 1 cup of mango and all the honey until the mixture becomes completely smooth. Divide into 4 glasses and refrigerate until ready to use. Rinse the blender.

2. Preheat the grill to medium-high heat. Mix the remaining cup of mango, ¼ cup water, ¼ cup vinegar, sultanas, olive oil, cayenne pepper, tomatoes and garlic in a microwave bowl. Cover with a piece of clear film and cook in the microwave until the tomatoes become soft, for about 3 minutes. Leave to cool slightly and pass in a blender. Transfer to a small bowl. Leave 2 tablespoons aside to garnish, turn the chicken into the remaining mixture.

3. Put the corn on the grill, cover and bake, turning it over if necessary, until it is burnt, about 10 minutes. Remove and keep warm.

4. Brush the grill over medium heat and brush the grills with a little oil. Turn the chicken legs into half the remaining sauce and ½ teaspoon of salt.

Put on the grill and cook until the cooking marks appear and the internal temperature reaches 75°C on an instantaneous thermometer, 8 to 10 minutes per side. Bart and sprinkle a few times with the remaining sauce while cooking.

5. While the chicken is cooking, beat the remaining 2 tablespoons of yogurt, the 2 tablespoons of sauce set aside, the remaining spoonful of vinegar, 1 tablespoon of water and ¼ teaspoon of salt in a large bowl. Mix the mixed salad with the carrots. Divide chicken, corn and salad into 4 serving dishes. Garnish the salad with the dressing set aside. Serve each plate with a mango smoothie.

Nutrition: Calories 346 Protein 56 Fat 45

Chinese Chicken Salad

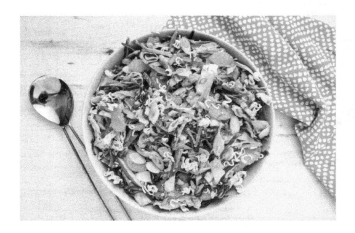

Preparation Time: 15 minutes

Cooking Time: 30 minutes

Servings: 4

Ingredients:

- For the chicken salad:
- 4 divided chicken breasts with skin and bones
- Olive oil of excellent quality
- Salt and freshly ground black pepper
- 500 g asparagus, with the ends removed and cut into three parts diagonally
- 1 red pepper, peeled
- Chinese condiment, recipe to follow

- 2 spring onions (both the white and the green part), sliced diagonally
- 1 tablespoon of white sesame seeds, toasted
- For Chinese dressing:
- 120 ml vegetable oil
- 60 ml of apple cider vinegar of excellent quality
- 60 ml soy sauce
- 1 ½ tablespoon of black sesame
- ½ tablespoon of honey
- 1 clove of garlic, minced
- ½ teaspoon of fresh peeled and grated ginger
- ½ tablespoon sesame seeds, toasted
- 60 g peanut butter
- 2 teaspoons of salt
- ½ teaspoons freshly ground black pepper

Directions:

1. For the chicken salad:
2. Heat the oven to 180°C (or 200°C for gas oven). Put the chicken breast on a baking tray and rub the skin with a little olive oil. Season freely with salt and pepper.
3. Brown for 35 to 40 minutes, until the chicken is freshly cooked. Let it cool down as long as it takes to handle it. Remove the meat from the bones,

remove the skin and chop the chicken into medium-sized pieces.

4. Blanch the asparagus in a pot of salted water for 3-5 minutes until tender. Soak them in water with ice to stop cooking. Drain them. Cut the peppers into strips the same size as the asparagus. In a large bowl, mix the chopped chicken, asparagus and peppers.

5. Spread the Chinese dressing on chicken and vegetables. Add the spring onions and sesame seeds, and season to taste. Serve cold or at room temperature.

6. For Chinese dressing:

7. Mix all ingredients and set aside until use.

Nutrition: Calories 222 Protein 28 Fat 10 Sugar 6

CONCLUSION

The things to watch out for when coming off keto are weight gain, bloating, more energy, and feeling hungry. The weight gain is nothing to freak out over; perhaps, you might not even gain any. It all depends on your diet, how your body processes carbs, and, of course, water weight. The length of your keto diet is a significant factor in how much weight you have lost, which is caused by the reduction of carbs. The bloating will occur because of the reintroduction of fibrous foods and your body getting used to digesting them again. The bloating van lasts for a few days to a few weeks. You will feel like you have more energy because carbs break down into glucose, which is the body's primary source of fuel. You may also notice better brain function and the ability to work out more.

Whether you have met your weight loss goals, your life changes, or you simply want to eat whatever you want again. You cannot just suddenly start consuming carbs again for it will shock your system. Have an idea of what you want to allow back into your consumption slowly. Be familiar with portion sizes and stick to that amount of carbs for the first few times you eat post-keto.

Start with non-processed carbs like whole grain, beans, and fruits. Start slow and see how your body responds before resolving to add carbs one meal at a time.

The ketogenic diet is the ultimate tool you can use to plan your future. Can you picture being more involved, more productive and efficient, and more relaxed and energetic? That future is possible for you, and it does not have to be a complicated process to achieve that vision. You can choose right now to be healthier and slimmer and more fulfilled tomorrow. It is possible with the ketogenic diet.

It does not just improve your physical health but your mental and emotional health as well. This diet improves your health holistically. Do not give up now as there will be quite a few days where you may think to yourself, "Why am I doing this?" and to answer that, simply focus on the goals you wish to achieve.

A good diet enriched with all the proper nutrients is our best shot of achieving an active metabolism and efficient lifestyle. A lot of people think that the Keto diet is simply for people who are interested in losing weight. You will find that it is quite the opposite. There are intense keto diets where only 5 percent of the diet comes from carbs, 20 percent is from protein, and 75 percent is from fat. But even a modified version of this which involves consciously choosing foods low in carbohydrate and high in healthy fats is good enough.

Thanks for reading this book. I hope it has provided you with enough insight to get you going. Don't put off getting started. The sooner you begin this diet, the sooner you'll start to notice an improvement in your health and well-being.

CPSIA information can be obtained
at www.ICGtesting.com
Printed in the USA
BVHW050433070421
604326BV00003B/154